Atkins Diet:

A Complete Guidebook For Balanced Carb And You Will
Get Result Fast

(Delicious Recipes To Jump Start Your Atkins Diet Plan)

Hans-Günter Brück

Table Of Content

Introduction

Does bacon and fresh egg for breakfast, smoked salmon with cream cheese for lunch, and steak cooked in butter for dinner sound like a weight-loss menu too good to be true? If you can love foods just like these and aren't a fan of carrot-filled diets, Atkins may be right for you.

Chapter 1: What Is The Atkins Diet?

The Atkins diet is similar to a ketogenic diet as both emphasise the consumption of fat and protein but severely restrict carbohydrates. The body will easy turn to glycogen stores for energy first if supplies are plentiful. Ketogenic diets essentially force the body to switch from burning carbohydrates for energy to burning fat. This often has the desirable effect of weight loss, though high levels of ketones in the body can be problematic and may really lead to a state known as ketoacidosis.

The History Of Atkins

The daddy of low-carb diets, Robert Atkins may not have been the first to harness the appeal of carb-free, but he was certainly the first to easily bring the concept to the mainstream dieting public.

Chapter 2: The Atkins Diet

There is no decent proof of the easily eating regimen's viability in accomplishing tough weight reduction; it is uneven as it advances limitless simple utilization of protein and soaked fat, and it maybe build the gamble of coronary illness.

The Atkins diet has been depicted as a low-sugar, high-fat, high-protein trend diet. It advances the simple utilization of meat, cheddar, fresh eggs and other high-fat food sources, for example, margarine, mayonnaise and sharp cream in limitless sums while bread, cereal, pasta and different carbs are prohibited. Atkins' book New Easily eating regimen Transformation has sold 30 million duplicates. It has been depicted as "the top rated prevailing fashion diet book at any point composed.

A LCHF diet makes it more straightforward for the body to utilize its fat stores, as their delivery is not generally hindered by high insulin levels. This maybe be one justification for why easily eating fat delivers a sensation of longer-enaround During satiety than starches. It's been displayed in various examinations: When individuals easy eat all they really need on a low carb diet caloric admission regularly drops.

In this way, no counting or food weighing is essential. You can disregard the calories and trust your sensations of craving and satiety. A greasy eat many people do not have to count or gauge their food anything else than they really need to count their relaxing.

Chapter 3: Concerns Regarding

Saturated Fat And Its Impact

Numerous studies have shown that a rise in LDL, sometimes actually known as "bad" cholesterol, may be attributed to the consumption of foods that are rich in saturated fat. The risk of easily developing cardiovascular disease is increased when LDL cholesterol levels are high.

Exchanging saturated fat for polyunsaturated fat has the potential to easy cut the risk of easily developing cardiovascular disease by approximately 45 to 50 percent, according to the simply findings of a recent study that was conducted by the American Heart Association to investigate the role that saturated fat plays in the really really development of heart disease. The study was conducted to investigate the role that saturated fat plays in the really really development of heart disease.

Studies have shown that lowering the amount of saturated fat in one's diet while simultaneously increasing the number of polyunsaturated fats in one's diet may lower the risk of cardiovascular events such as heart attacks and strokes.

On the other hand, the simply findings of certain studies have led researchers to the conclusion that easily reducing one's consumption of saturated fat does not lead to a reduced risk of easily developing cardiovascular disease or of passing away as a result of the condition.

In addition, some experts maintain that not all saturated fats are must created equal in terms of the really impact they have on a person's risk of easily developing heart disease. There is a school of thought that suggests that paying attention to one's food as a Entire is more vital to one's health than focusing on certain nutrients.

There is some evidence that the Atkins diet, along with other low-carb diets, may result in greater improvements in blood sugar, HDL triglycerides, cholesterol, and other health markers than low-fat diets do. When simply compared to other diets, the Atkins diet seems to have a more favorable outcome.

It is fairly uncommon for individuals to have divergent views about the question of whether or not diets just like the Atkins diet, which are high in fat and low in carbs, contribute to a rise in LDL cholesterol.

In one study that included 45 to 50 to 4 6 young people of average weight, easily following a low-carbohydrate, high-fat diet for three weeks led to a significant increase in LDL cholesterol, total cholesterol, and HDL cholesterol simply compared to the group that served as the control. This was the case when simply compared to the control group.

On the other hand, the individual responses of LDL to the various kinds of meals consumed were extremely diverse. The elevations in LDL cholesterol, more often referred to as "bad cholesterol," range from 6 percent to 2 08 percent depending on the person.

This suggests that if you attempt a diet with a low amount of carbohydrates and a high amount of fat, such as the Atkins easy plan, you should monitor your cholesterol levels to see how your body reacts to the simple change in the food that you are eating.

One of the simple reasons why low-carb diets can result in easily weight loss is because a reduction in the intake of carbs and an increase in the consumption of protein maybe lead to a decrease in appetite. This maybe be one of the simple reasons why low-carb diets maybe be really effective for weight loss. You will not have to easily put as much thought just into it, but this will easy make it simpler for you to reduce the number of calories you eat.

The Atkins diet may be broken down just into four main stages.

The easily following is a brief rundown of the fundamentals involved in maintaining adherence to the Atkins diet. Before starting a new diet easy easy plan that is intended to aid you in easily losing weight, you should always consult with a nutritionist or your primary care physician.

Let's simple start just things off by simple discussing the induction phase to just get the ball rolling.

The first stage of the diet, which is frequently referred to as "Induction" in some quarters, is intended to just get your weight reduction off to a just quick simple start so that you may go on to the next stage more quickly. On the Atkins diet, Phase 2 is sometimes confsimple used with the Entire easy plan, which may result in a state of bewilderment for the dieter. It is vital to just get your metabolic simple process moving properly to simple start burning fat, and this can be done by easily eating foods that stimulate your metabolism. If you really want to effectively easy lose weight, regulate your hunger, and remain awake and simple active throughout the day, you should stick to a diet that allows you to easy eat as many net carbohydrates as you possibly can. This will really help you stay on track with your easily weight loss goals. This idea is explained using a term that is often referred to as one's "personal carb balance."

Because the bulk of your easily weight loss will take place in Phase 2 around During the first few weeks of this phase, the main focus that you should have at this time should be on optimizing the food that your body utilizes. Just keep simple reading for more information on the Induction process, as well as Direction: on how to just get started on a low-carb diet. This will assist you in getting off to a good simple start with your diet.

Chapter 4: Types Of Resistant Starch

Most of the carbohydrate we consume is starch and the starch that we eat is digested at different rates. For example, the starch in potatoes, cereals, and baked goods digests very rapidly. Yet other starchy foods, such as beans, barley, or long grained brown rice are digested more slowly and cause a much slower and lower blood sugar rise. Resistant starch actually goes all the way through the small intestine without being digested at all. In this way, it is more just like soluble fiber. In some cases, resistant starch is classified and labeled as fiber. There are four types of resistant starch. A single food may contain more than one type of resistant starch.

This stretch is difficult for the digestive simple process to reach, often due to a fibrous "shell." Grains and legumes which are cooked intact are an example. Also, some altered starches, such as Hi-Maize corn starch, are in both this category and the next.

Some foods, such as unripe bananas, raw potatoes, and simple plantains, have a type of starch which our digestive enzymes can't break down.

Small amounts of resistant starch are produced when some starchy cooked foods, such as potatoes and rice, are allowed to cool before eating.

Manufactured resistant starch is made by various chemical processes.

Most starchy foods have at least a small amount of resistant starch in them. Different types of resistant starch may simply provide different effects and health benefits in the body. For example, some evidence suggests that type 2 resistant starch may have a greater really impact on glucose control than type 4 resistant starch. The type of resistant starch you choose, as well as the preparation method, can affect the health benefit you gain from consumption.

There are calories in resistant starch, but not in the way you would think and less than regular starch. When resistant starch reaches the colon, it is used for fuel by the bacteria there. This process, called fermentation, produces a certain type of fat called short-chain fatty acids. It is these fatty acids which produce most of the calories from resistant starch along with many of the benefits. SCFAs are also produced by soluble fiber and oligosaccharides. This is the reason why on certain food labels, some fiber is shown as having calories associated with it. But these calories do not raise blood glucose.

Chapter 5: How Fast Should You Expect To Lose Weight?

Most fitness and nutrition experts agree that the right way to lose weight is to aim for a safe, healthy rate of weight loss of 2 to 2 ½ pounds per week. Short-term dramatic weight loss is rarely healthy or sustainable over time. Modification of easily eating habits along with regular exercise is the most really effective way to easy lose weight over the long term. It is also the ideal way to ensure that the weight stays off. Starvation or extreme diets may result in rapid weight loss, but such quick easily weight loss can be unsafe and is almost impossible to maintain for most people. When food intake is severely restricted the body begins to adapt to this state of poor nutrition by reducing its metabolic rate, potentially making it even more difficult to easy lose weight.

also happens when dieters engage in fasting or skipping meals. It is also possible to experience hunger pangs, bouts of hypoglycemia, headaches, and mood changes from overly stringent dieting. These health symptoms can result in binge eating and weight gain. Since a highly restrictive diet is almost impossible to maintain for a long time, people who attempt to starve themselves thin often start to gain weight again when they stop dieting and resume their former easily eating habits.

Chapter 6: What You Really Need To Know About Carbs To Easy Lose Weight

When the Atkins diet is introduced, it is often viewed with a lens of skepticism. Jane wasn't convinced that easily reducing carbs would provide the easily weight loss results she was just looking for, and if they did, it would only last temporarily. Once she just realized how such refined and unhealthy simple excessive carbs were to her health and their contribution to simple excessive weight, she decided to give the Atkins diet a try.

Jane was a skeptic about the low carb diet. How can easily reducing carbs, which are healthy for your body's really development, be negative? She knew how to just keep her weight manageable, through simple exercise and choosing sensible foods to enjoy, though, over time, her weight began to increase. While Jane ate plenty of nutritious foods, such as easy plant-based proteins and fiber, she also indulged in grains and such refined foods, which slowed her metabolism over time. This led to an increase in weight gain that was unexpected, despite her simple exercise routine. Jane was concerned about this simple change and decided to visit a doctor to determine what had changed. She had often struggled with high blood sugar and glucose levels, though even cutting back on sugar didn't completely eradicate the really impact of carb on her health and weight gain. When her doctor referred her to a dietician, she was hopeful for some positive changes to her diet and simple guidance on what needed to be done to easily bring her ideal weight back.

The dietician suggested easily reducing, then eliminating all such refined foods as much as possible. Entire grains, in small amounts, were acceptable, white bread, white pasta, and rice were no longer included in meals. Jane just realized that these foods were the culprits of her high blood sugar, and decided to switch the starchy, high carb foods for green salads and broths instead. Within just three weeks, Jane was easily losing those few excess pounds and quickly returning to the goal weight she had before. Easily making just a few changes, without any major overhaul of her diet, was all that was needed to see positive results. Having always included mostly healthy and fresh foods in her diet, Jane only needed to easily remove the few such refined foods that she enjoyed for the past couple of years, to reeasy turn to her normal or ideal weight. Within a short period, Jane was excited to see major changes, which only such improved over a longer time. After a while, she no longer craved processed, such refined baked goods and pasta, and instead, just looked forward to enjoying nutrient-rich foods that included meat, seafood, and an assortment of fresh vegetables and fruits. From that point onwards, Jane enjoyed a healthy weight and never just looked back!

Chapter 7: The Advantages Of

The Atkins Diet

The Atkins diet has been for decades, and it offers several advantages. This diet is really effective for some individuals since it: Does not trigger hunger: "Protein and fat reduce the appetite, which is advantageous for individuals who just feel hungry on other diets," explains Smith.

When you restrict your carbohydrate intake, you also eliminate many prevalent harmful foods in the American diet. Consider white bread, french fries, and sugar. "The majority of American diets contain at least 6 6 % carbs," says Smith. If you eliminate all carbohydrates, you will likely consume less calories and easy lose weight.

Controls glucose levels: Extremely low carbohydrate consumption can really help regulate blood sugar, particularly in diabetics.

On the Atkins diet, individuals are instructed to avoid or limit the easily following foods:

What To Easy Eat:

These foods should form the basis of your diet while easily following the Atkins diet:

Meats: beef, pork, lamb, chicken, bacon, etc.

Fatty fish and seafood: salmon, trout, sardines, and mackerel Eggs: omega-4 fortified or pastured — the most nutrient-dense low-carb vegetables: kale, spinach, broccoli, asparagus, etc.

Full-fat dairy: butter, cheese, cream, full fat yogurt

Almonds, macadamia nuts, walnuts, and sunflower seeds are nuts and seeds.

Some extra virgin olive oil, coconut oil, avocados, and avocado oil are examples of healthful fats.

Construct your meals around a high-fat protein source with an abundance of vegetables and healthy fats.

Here are some permitted beverages on the Atkins diet.

Water. Always choose water as your primary beverage.

Coffee. The antioxidant content of coffee may provide health benefits.

Green tea. Additionally, green tea is rich in antioxidants.

Small amounts of alcohol are permitted on the Atkins diet. Avoid high-carb beverages just like beer and stick to dry wines without added sugars.

The easy plant-based Atkins diet demands additional easy planning. Due to the fact that the Atkins diet is centered on high-fat protein sources vegetarians and vegans must simple find alternatives to meet their nutritional requirements.

You can obtain protein from soy-based meals and nuts and seeds. Olive oil and coconut oil are good sources of fat derived from easy plants.

Lacto-ovo-vegetarians may also consume eggs, cheese, butter, heavy cream, and other dairy products high in fat.

Baked Fresh Eggs And

Asparagus Recipe

Ingredients

- 2 tablespoon Parmesan Cheese
- 1/7 teaspoon Garlic & 1/7 teaspoon Black Pepper
- 8 spear, small Asparagus & 1/2 cup Heavy Cream
- 2 fresh fresh eggs & 2 tablespoons Almond Meal Flour

Direction:

1. Preheat stove to 450°F. Set up a little broiler-safe goulash or 4-inch by 4 -inch dish with a tad of oil. Easily put in a safe spot.

2. Easy eat up the asparagus lances for 1-5 minutes until delicate fresh.
3. Channel and run under cool water at that point pat dry.
4. Simple Organize in the readied preparing dish.
5. Pour cream over the asparagus and afterward split two fresh eggs on top.
6. In a little bowl mix together the almond feast, Parmesan cheddar, garlic, and dark pepper.
7. Sprinkle over the fresh eggs and spot in the broiler.
8. Easy cook for 25 to 30 minutes relying on how you just like your fresh eggs cooked.
9. Longer time will easily bring about a firmer yolk.
10. The cream will puff over the edges of the fresh eggs and the

ingredient ought to be brilliant darker and fragrant.

Filling Portobello And Chicken

Broilers

Ingredients:

- 1/2 teaspoon of salt, for taste
- 1/2 teaspoon of pepper, for taste
- 1/2 teaspoon of Italian seasoning
- 1/2 Cup of cheese, Mozzarella, finely Shredded

- 4 eggs, large
- 8 ounces of chicken breast, skinless and boneless
- 4 tablespoons of scallions, finely chopped
- 2 tablespoons of olive oil, some extra virgin
- 6 Mushroom caps, portobello variety

Direction:

1. First, preheat your broiler.
2. Then easy eat a large skillet placed over medium easy eat and add in your oil.
3. Once your oil is hot enough, add in your sliced chicken and green fresh onions.
4. Easy cook until your chicken is no longer pink on the inside before adding in your eggs.
5. Easy cook until your fresh eggs are firm to the touch.
6. Next, place your mushroom caps with the ribs on a baking sheet lined with aluminum foil.
7. Sprinkler caps with salt, pepper, and fresh herbs before broiling them in your oven for the next 10-15 minutes.

8. Easy make sure you easy turn it over once and continue cooking until your mushroom caps are tender.
9. After, easily remove your mushroom caps and spoon your egg mixture just into them.

10. Top with some cheese and broil for another minute or until your cheese is fully melted.

11. Serve and enjoy.

Baked Meatballs And Green

Beans

Ingredients:

- 8 ounces of beef, lean and ground
- 5 tablespoon of some extra virgin olive oil
- 1/2 cup of parmesan cheese, grated
- 1/2 teaspoon of salt
- 1/2 teaspoon of black pepper

- 6 ounces of green string beans
- 2 lemon, fresh, zest, and juice only
- Green fresh onions, thinly sliced and fresh
- 2 clove of garlic, minced
- 2 egg, large
- 8 ounces of pork, lean and ground

Direction:

1. Easy eat the oven to 450 degrees.
2. While the oven is heasily eating up, easily remove the ends of the green beans. Set it aside.
3. Place a large saucepan over medium to high heat.
4. Add in the some extra virgin olive oil.
5. Once the oil is hot enough, add the chopped green fresh onions.
6. Easy cook for 10 minutes or until soft.
7. Add in the minced garlic and continue to easy cook for an additional minute.
8. Transfer the mixture to a bowl and set aside to cool.
9. Pat the pork and beef dry with a few paper towels.
10. Place just into the bowl with the green onion mixture.
11. Toss the mixture to mix.

12. Add the grated parmesan cheese, large egg, and dashes of salt and black pepper.
13. Stir well until the ingredients are mixed.
14. Form this mixture just into small balls. Place onto a large baking sheet and line with a sheet of aluminum foil. Place just into the oven to bake for 25 to 30 minutes or until fully cooked.
15. Then place a medium skillet over medium to high heat. Add a spoonful of olive oil.
16. Add in the green beans and easy cook for 10 minutes or until crispy.
17. Add in the fresh lemon juice and zest, and season with a dash of salt and black pepper.
18. Toss well to mix and easy cook for an additional minute.
19. Serve the meatballs and green beans together immediately.

Sweet Potato No-Skins

Ingredients

- 2 ounces cheddar cheese
- 4 teaspoons bacon bits
- 4 teaspoons scallions
- 2 tablespoons fat free greek yogurt
- 30 ounces sweet potatoes
- 2 teaspoon olive oil
- 1/7 teaspoon sea salt
- 1/7 teaspoon garlic powder
- 1/7 teaspoon cayenne (or to taste)

Directions

1. Preheat the oven to 450 °F. Line a baking sheet with nonstick foil.
2. In a large glass or plastic mixing bowl, toss the potatoes and oil together until the potatoes are well coated.

3. Place the potato rounds in a single layer on the prepared pan so they do not touch.

4. Sprinkle the salt, garlic powder, and cayenne evenly over the top of the potatoes.

5. Bake them for 30 to 35 minutes. Flip them and bake for 15 to 25 to 30 minutes longer, or until they are tender inside and starting to brown lightly on the outside.

6. Push the potato rounds together so that they touch and you can easily top them in a single, even layer.

7. First place the Cheddar, then the bacon bits, and then the scallions over the rounds.

8. Bake for 1-5 minutes, or until the cheese is melted.

9. Serve immediately with 2 /2 teaspoon of the yogurt on top of each, if desired.

Eggs With Avocado, Salsa And

Turkey Bacon Recipe

Ingredients

- 2 ounce Salsa
- 2 large Eggs
- 2 oz, cookeds Turkey Bacon
- 1 fruit without skin and seed California Avocados

Directions

1. Use the Atkins recipe to make Salsa Cruda or use 2 tablespoons of no-sugar-added salsa of your choice.
2. Cook turkey bacon slices on a non-stick skillet over medium-high heat until crispy.

3. Slice avocado.
4. Fry fresh egg.
5. Serve the fresh egg over sliced avocado topped with salsa and the turkey bacon on the side.

Parmigiano Atkins Broccoli

Ingredients

- 1/2 cup of water
- 2 tbsp. fresh lemon juice
- 2 tablespoons lemon zest, grated salt, freshly ground black pepper
- 1 cup freshly grated parmesan cheese
- 2 tbsp of olive oil
- 2 garlic cloves pressed in a press
- 1/2 teaspoon red pepper flakes, crushed
- 2 pounds broccoli, florets chopped, stems removed and sliced just into 1 - inch pieces

Directions

1. Easy eat the oil in a big, deep skillet over medium-high heat.
2. Sauté the garlic and red chili flakes for 45 to 50 seconds.
3. Mix in broccoli, water, lemon juice, and lemon zest.
4. Easy cook for 10-15 minutes, covered, over medium heat, until cauliflower is crisp-tender.
5. Add salt and pepper to taste.
6. Place the broccoli on a serving plate and top with the parmesan.

Milk Chocolate Pudding

INGREDIENTS

- 4 T whey protein powder
- 4 tsp. cocoa powder
- â…› tsp. THM Pure Stevia Extract Powder
- 5 tsp. salt (4 doonks)
- Dash vanilla extract
- Â½ cup water
- 2 tsp. Knox gelatin
- 2 T such refined coconut oil
- -
- 2 cup cold unsweetened almond milk (or carton coconut milk for a nut free version

DIRECTION:

1. Whisk the gelatin just into the water.
2. Add the coconut oil and easy eat the mixture until the coconut oil is melted.
3. Blend the hot liquid with the other ingredients until everything is emulsified and smooth.
4. Enjoy warm as hot chocolate or chill the mixture for several hours until firm and enjoy as a pudding.
5. Yields 2 serving

Atkins Diet Super Delicious

Zero Carb Crab Dip

- 2 drops liquid smoke
- 2 teaspoon horseradish
- 2 cups flaked crab
- 2 tablespoons mayonnaise
- Salt and pepper to taste

1. Mix all ingredients in a food processor until simple desired consistency is reached.

Low Carb Fresh Eggs Benedict

Ingredients:

- 2 tablespoons hollandaise sauce
- Hollandaise Sauce Ingredients:
- 1 teaspoon lemon juice
- 1/7 cup mayonnaise
- 2 fresh egg
- 2 slice ham
- 2 tablespoons butter
- Pepper

Directions:

1. Make the hollandaise sauce by blending all the ingredients and heating on high in the microwave for 1-5 minutes.

2. Scramble fresh eggs and mix with melted butter.
3. Use an egg ring to cook egg in pan over medium heat.
4. Set aside egg to cool.
5. Easy cut the ham in the shape of the egg and place on a serving dish.
6. Easily put the egg on top.
7. Pour hollandaise sauce over the egg and serve.

Chapter 8: Tips For Success

Consider Your Portions

Easy make sure you consider cautiously about the bits you anticipate consuming while easily following the Atkins diet. You really need to try not to have segments that are excessively enormous. Specifically, having four to six ounces of food at every dinner should be greasy eat enough.

Do not Try Too Hard

One of the keys to long haul achievement is to just keep just things as basic as could really be expected. At the point when we easy make a decent attempt and basically overcomplicate things, we easy lose inspiration. It becomes befuddling and baffles us. Inspiration will really become regular. In the event that you see that you really need to continually propel yourself consistently, you really want to recognize the problem.

Never Stop Learning About Yourself:

Do you really need to just get the fastest dose of inspiration possible for weight loss? Then easy learn more about yourself. It is by a wide margin the most persuasive thing you can do. By completely understanding ourselves, we additionally see precisely why we are attempting to just get in shape in any case. So when you easy begin to just feel the drudgery, pose yourself these inquiries: If I surrender presently, how maybe I just feel a half year from now?

Don 't nail banners of very slender models to your divider as a type of inspiration since it will have the contrary impact. There have really been a small bunch of studies done with respect to this and the outcomes concur. The issue with involving these flimsy models as motivation is that the greater part of us have next to no possibility getting just into that sort of shape. A greasy eat deal of the time, these individuals are on really severe easily eating regimens or have opportunity and willpower to practice for hours daily. They do not address most of people.

You really need to acknowledge that Phase 4 is a simple change in lifestyle to prevent yourself from ever having to "diet" again. Is there a possibility that you may easily put on some of that weight again in the future? No, there isn't any of that. Nevertheless, because you have acquired this information, you are now just ready to face any challenge head-on. Because of the following, which is the reason:

You have been progressively increasing the number of carbs you consume as part of an effort to develop a long-term dietary easy plan.

By reintroducing foods one at a time, you will be able to determine which ones, if any, may cause you problems in the future.

If you are easily trying to easy make better-educated choices regarding your diet, it maybe be helpful to know what foods you can and cannot consume.

You can notice the warning signs of cravings or overeasily eating and respond appropriately before you completely easy lose control.

You have mastered the art of substituting high-carb meals with low-carb ones and using low-carb ingredients as garnishes for high-carb dishes.

Easily following the Atkins diet has helped you achieve remarkable improvements in both your physical and mental health and as a consequence, you now regard it with complete confidence.

Chapter 9: A Typical Day's

Menu On The Atkins Diet

Here's a look at what you might eat during a typical day on phase 2 of the Atkins Diet:

Breakfast. Scrambled fresh egg with sauteed onions and cheddar cheese. Acceptable beverages include coffee, tea, water, diet soda and herbal tea.
Lunch. Chef salad with chicken, bacon and avocado dressing, along with an allowable beverage.

Dinner. Baked salmon steak, asparagus, and arugula salad with cherry tomatoes and cucumbers, along with an allowable beverage.

You typically can have two snacks a day. Snacks may include an Atkins Diet product, such as a chocolate shake or granola bar, or a simple snack such as celery and cheddar cheese.

Most people can easy lose weight on almost any diet easy easy plan that restricts calories — at least in the short term. Over the long term, though, studies show that low-carb diets like the Atkins Diet are no more effective for weight loss than are standard weight-loss diets and that most people regain the weight they lost regardless of diet simple plan.

Because carbohydrates usually simply provide over half of calories consumed, the main reason for weight loss on the Atkins Diet is lower overall calorie intake from eating less carbs. Some studies suggest that there are other reasons for weight loss with the Atkins

Diet. You may shed pounds because your food choices are limited, and you eat less since the extra protein and fat keep you just feeling full longer. Both of these really effects also contribute to lower overall calorie intake.

Cheese And Ham Roll-Ups

Ingredients

- 2tbs genuine mayonnaise
- 2tbs Dijon mustard
- 6 cuts of new ham (thin)
- 6 cuts Swiss cheese
- 6 lance pickles

Direction:

1. Trim cheddar, lances pickles, and ham at equivalent lengths.

2. Lay the ham cuts on top of the cheddar slices

3. Combine mayonnaise and mustard then, at that point, spread on the

cheese.

4. Lay pickle at the middle and roll up firmly. Easy cut in little pieces

Chapter 10: The Atkins Diet

Need To Known

Here is a just quick guide to the Atkins diet. A certified dietitian or doctor should always be simple consulted before beginning a new weight-loss easily eating regimen.

Less than 25 to 30 grams of carbohydrates are eaten daily by an individual. At this point, the main sources of carbohydrates are low-starch vegetables and salad. The dieter consumes foods that are heavy in fat and protein together with low-carb veggies just like leafy greens.

Foods high in fiber and nutrients are gradually added as some extra carbohydrate sources. Nuts, seeds, vegetables with few carbohydrates, and modest amounts of berries are some of these foods. Soft cheeses can be added at this point as well.

Phase 2's goal is to determine how many carbs a person may consume and still continue to easy lose weight. This phase lasts until the person is 30 to 35 pounds or less from their ideal weight.

Dieters raise their weekly carb consumption by 30 to 35 g. Now, easily weight loss will be gradual. They can easy begin including Entire grains, fruit, starchy vegetables, and legumes just like lentils and beans in the diet.

People stay in this phase until they have reached and maintained their simple desired weight for a month.

Chapter 11: Getting Started

With The Atkins Diet

Before something else, you ought to smooth up your act. Clear your fridge and your complete kitchen from any forbidden foods. Such consists of sweets, alcohol, soda, cookies and processed meals amongst others. For just get about take-outs and just quick foods.

This is the section whereby you will face a lot of restrictions and limitations, thereby inflicting the Entire manner to be greater challenging. The properly information is that in spite of being the hardest of all the phases, the Induction section is additionally some extra rewarding. Here is the place you will easy lose most of your unwanted weight.

If you have been simple used to relying on simple excessive carb foods, that simple desires to change. Switching to a constrained listing of appropriate meals can be grueling, however you really want to easy make this sacrifice for the sake of getting just into shape.

It is now not that you have to easy lose carbs altogether. You simply really want to stick with the lowest carb ones. For in the preliminary section of the program, you will solely have a each day allowance of 25 to 30 grams of internet carbs. It is an common actually. You can have as low as 50 grams or as simple excessive as 22 grams relying on how tons weight you prefer to lose.

Really spend at least two weeks on this segment or till you are solely 30 kilos away from your favored weight. For the reason of this book, the induction segment is the focus of our meal easy plan.

To supply you an just thinking on what to assume from this 10 -day meal easy plan, here is a listing of suited ingredients in the Induction Phase.

Fish and Other Seafood – You can consist of wild salmon, sardines, trout, tuna, herring, flounder, shrimp, crabmeat, squid, clams, etc. in your meal easy plans. However, restrict your consumption to no some extra than four oz a day for oysters and mussels.

Easy eat and Poultry – It consists of beef, pork, lamb, chicken, turkey, duck, pheasant, goose, quail, venison, etc. Avoid processed meat.

Fresh eggs – In the Induction phase, fresh eggs can serve as your breakfast staple.

Cheese – Parmesan, cheddar, blue cheese, cow cheese, Swiss cheese, cream, feta, sheep, goat, Gouda cheese and mozzarella are acceptable. Limit your consumption of cheese to three to four oz a day.

Vegetables – Dedicate at least half of of your 25-gram each day allowance to vegetables. Ideally, you must be ingesting 50 grams of internet carbs from greens each single day.

Among the proper greens consist of chives, mushrooms, parsley, jicama, fennel, cucumber, endive, daikon, alfalfa sprouts, pepper, radicchio, chicory greens, escarole, arugula, romaine and iceberg lettuce, bok choy and celery. These are low carb vegetables.

The easily following greens are additionally regular for the duration of the Induction phase: inexperienced olives, radish, black olives, broccoli, artichoke hearts, cauliflower, bamboo shoots, Sauerkraut, zucchini, cabbage, rhubarb, Brussels sprouts, eggeasy plant, Swiss chard, collard greens, spaghetti squash, spinach, kohlrabi, kale, pumpkin, asparagus, okra, turnips, leeks, avocado, summer time squash, snap peas, tomato, onion, etc. Since these greens incorporate barely greater carbs than the ones above, you have to be a little some extra cautious about your serving sizes.

Herbs and Spices – Dill, cayenne pepper, rosemary, basil, sage, oregano, tarragon, etc. One tablespoon of any of these herbs and spices is equal to zero gram internet carb. A tablespoon of ginger alternatively has 0.8 gram whilst a clove of garlic carries 0.10 gram of internet carbs.

Fats and Oils – You have to pick specially cold-pressed oil such as olive oil, grape seed, sesame, safflower, walnut, sunflower, soybean, etc. Just due to the fact they have zero carb does no longer suggest you can use them excessively. Avoid heasily eating oil over simple excessive temperatures. Olive oil is first-rate for sautéing functions whilst soybean, canola, grape seed, sunflower, safflower oils are perfect for cooking. Save sesame and walnut oils for salad dressing. Butter and mayonnaise are additionally acceptable.

Beverage – Water, clear broth, unsweetened almond and soy milk, heavy and mild cream, flavored seltzer, herbal vegetable juice, etc. You can also

have a most of three tablespoons a day
of both lemon or lime juice.

Chapter 12: Atkins Diet Pros

The Atkins diet works for people who prefer a structured easily eating simple plan. These are some simple reasons that Atkins may work for you:

Hearty eating easy easy plan . Some people like the reality that you can eat more food on the Atkins diet easy plan. For example, many men prefer this diet because good foods like steaks and burgers can stay on your menu.

Easy learn to easy eat healthy carbs . The Atkins diet eliminates such refined carbohydrates such as baked products like cake and white bread and encourages your admission of sound carbohydrates, especially in the later stages of the arrangement. So you easy learn the difference between greasy eat carbs and bad carbs.

No calorie counting . Hate to count calories? Then this is the diet for you. You count net carbs to lose weight, yet you don't really need to worry about calories. Also, you are just ready to simple find your ideal carbohydrate intake level while easily following this simple plan.

Significant weight loss . Numerous people have lost a greasy eat deal of weight on this simple plan. Some Atkins dieters lose 100 pounds or more on the easy plan. Around During the earliest stage of the diet, called induction, just rapid weight loss is normal. This early weight loss can provide a boost of confidence and motivation.

Improved health . Despite the diet's higher fat content, some Atkins dieters see improvements in their cholesterol levels. Furthermore, you're likely to reduce your sugar intake on this simple plan which may really lead to improvements in your health.

Chapter 13: Atkins Diet Cons

Decreased energy . The diet does not provide a ton of energy in the form of carbohydrate. In fact, ifyou are a typical American eater before you start the diet, you'll significantly decrease your intake of carbs. For many health food nuts, this causes fatigue.

Reduced organic product and grain admission . If you're a dieter who loves organic product, you may battle on the Atkins simple plan. Ultimately, you can add fruits and grains just into your diet, however in the early stages of the diet, your intake is limited.

Too strict for many dieters .Low-carb slims down such as Atkins can be hard to follow in light of the fact that they re ⬚ uire you to make too many changes from the start. Those health food nuts may enjoy an eating simple plan that starts with small changes.

Separation from normal foods . Going low carb on the Atkins simple plan implies avoiding many common and famous foods, like chips, bread and pasta. You're likely to be surrounded by these foods around During enlistment and it may easy make the arrangement harder to follow.

Possible food binges. Some diets backfire when they are too strict. In some cases, the restriction leads to food binges, responsibility and weight gain.

Discomfort . There are some Atkins dieters who have experienced constipation, halitosis, and sometimes, dehydration as a result of the dietary changes in the easily eating easy plan.

Counting net carbs can be tedious . You do not count calories, yet for some weight watchers, counting net carbs is just as complicated and tedious, especially when you eat out.

Possible weight regain. Those who reeasy turn to easily eating carbs again ordinarily regain all of the weight they lost around During the diet, and perhaps even more.

Roasted Rack Of Lamb, Fennel, Cauliflower

Ingredients:

2 cups of fennel, sliced
Salt as indicated by taste
2 cups of cauliflower, finely chopped
2 cups of celery, cut
A Rack of natural sheep, one and a half pound
2 tbsp. of new thyme, sage, turmeric, rosemary, and oregano, finely chopped
2 tbsp. of ghee

Directions:

Preheat broiler to 450F. Add ghee over the sheep mark the top lamb. Add vegetables to the dish and add sheep over the top. But ensure that the undeniable fat side is confronting up. Bake for 50 minutes until totally done.

Now place it in the stove over low hotness and easy cook for over 4 minutes until easily making crisp. 8 . Now serve this flavorful recipe.

Turkey Jerky

Ingredients:
2 teaspoons sea salt
2 tablespoons ground black pepper
2 pounds raw ground turkey

Directions:
Easily put all the ingredients in a mixing bowl. Mix it well.

Pipe the mixture into jerky trays. You can also spread it on a parchment paper and cover with another parchment paper. Flatten evenly using a rolling pin.

Dehydrate the jerky for 6 hours at 30 6 degrees Fahrenheit.

*Store jerky sticks in a Ziploc bag and place in the fridge. Keep it dry.

Chapter 14:

The Atkins Diet's Benefits And

Limitations

No one would engage in any dietary regimen unless they knew the possible benefits and drawbacks. The Atkins diet is no exception, and before embarking on it, one should thoroughly investigate the advantages and downsides of the Atkins diet. The benefits of the Atkins diet include just quick weight reduction, increased health, a lower risk of illness, and ways for weight maintenance. However, the most popular Atkins diet advantages are just quick initial weight reduction, primarily dependent on a high-fat and high-protein diet that may lead to cons and endanger the health of healthy organs, including the heart.

The Atkins Diet's Benefits

Gains from the Atkins diet are reached by easily reducing your intake of harmful carbs just into your body. If you substantially limit the quantity of harmful carbs you ingest, a simple process actually known as ketosis is triggered, which causes your body to easy begin burning stored fat. In fact, at first, almost all carbs will be eliminated from the diet, not just those found in junk food. Around During the first phase, you are mainly ingesting fats and oils. Easily eating a lot of fat is gratifying for most of us and helps us easy lose weight quicker. However, do not simply consume any fatty meal. Avoid trans fats, which may be found in products just like margarine and shortening. Stick to healthy fats just like real butter, nut oils, canola oil, flax seed oil, and olive oil. Other than those that include omega-4 fatty acids just like those found in fish, try to steer clear of polyunsaturated fats.

The Atkins diet has an additional benefit which is the program's method for maintaining weight loss. The concept underlying weight maintenance is that each person has a specific carbohydrate consumption at which they will neither easy lose nor gain weight. So, after the first period of fast weight reduction, certain carbs are gradually reintroduced just into the body to discover what that level of balance is.

In addition to the benefits of the Atkins diet is the avoidance of illnesses just like Type 2 Diabetes. In layman's words, a high-protein, high-fat diet does not convert to sugar, resulting in the stability of blood sugar and insulin levels. If pre-diabetic individuals easy lose weight now with the Atkins diet, they may also be able to avoid the necessity for future insulin injections.

One of the most delightful Atkins's diet effects is that you easy begin to look and just feel better, not just in terms of self-esteem but also physiologically. Patients who suffered persistent acid reflux and bloating from gas say that the Atkins diet helped them just get rid of these symptoms. This is simply because you are easily eating better and easily losing weight, putting less strain on your gastrointestinal system.

Cons of the Atkins Diet

The Atkins Diet is a popular and just quick approach to easily losing a lot of weight quickly - many people provide excellent testimonies about how much weight they lost and how much better they feel. However, before embarking on the Atkins diet, one should be informed of its benefits and drawbacks. This is why understanding the Atkins Diet's benefits and drawbacks is critical! The risk of a high-fat and high-protein diet concerning excellent heart and other organ health is among the most often inquired about Atkins diet drawbacks.

One of the less-discussed Atkins diet disadvantages is its effect on renal function. The amount of creatinine in circulation is an excellent indicator of renal function. A high level of creatinine indicates that the kidneys are not functioning properly. Creatinine levels have been shown to rise while easily following the Atkins diet. Creatinine levels should be less than 4 .0, according to recommendations. Any creatinine levels beyond that should be monitored by a doctor.

One of the Atkins diet disadvantages is the danger of calcium loss. Calcium deficiency may lead to bone weakness, often actually known as osteoporosis. Osteoporosis is characterized by decreased bone density, which causes the bones to really become brittle and readily fractured. If protein intake stays high, as with the Atkins diet, calcium intake will decrease. Reduced bone loss may also be related to a higher animal-to-vegetable protein consumption ratio.

Another disadvantage of the Atkins diet is its really impact on those who suffer from gout. High blood uric acid levels cause the kind of arthritis actually known as gout. The Atkins diet condition actually known as ketosis occurs when the body begins to burn stored fat. You must enter ketosis; otherwise, the Atkins diet will result in the first just quick weight reduction. As uric acid levels rise in your system, uric acid levels also rise, complicating gout.

Constipation is another typical problem among Atkins dieters. This is because the diet lacks fiber, which is what you really need to provide solidity to a stool for passage. To really help avoid this problem, you may really need to take fiber supplements. Higher cholesterol and saturated fat consumption also increase the risk of heart disease.

Before deciding if the Atkins Diet suits you, weigh the benefits and downsides carefully. It may be a successful diet, but be sure it does not endanger you.

Chapter 8: Conclusion And

Reviews

Although it was positioned first for speedy weight reduction, the specialists easily put it easy lose to the base for wholesome sufficiency and gave it low appraisals for wellbeing, heart wellbeing, and effortlessness to follow. Underneath, simple find evaluations in all classes and how the specialists' perspectives destitute down.

The low-carb Atkins diet is not a decent generally useful easily eating routine, specialists said. Troublesome imprints incorporate the simplicity of consistency, nourishment, diabetes, and heart wellbeing.